Plum Tree Guide for Beginners

Harvesting and Utilizing Plum Fruit

By

Brogan Callum

Table of Contents

CHAPTER 1

Introduction

1.1 What Are Plum Trees?

Plum trees, scientifically classified as members of the Prunus genus within the Rosaceae family, represent an esteemed and diverse group of deciduous fruit-bearing trees cherished for their delicious fruits and ornamental value. These trees, with their characteristic blossoms and succulent fruits, hold a prominent place in horticulture, history, and culinary traditions worldwide.

Botanical Essence and Diversity: Plum trees exhibit remarkable diversity in their size, shape, and fruit characteristics. They belong to a larger group that encompasses various cultivars, hybrids, and species, each possessing unique attributes in terms of fruit color, flavor, texture, and adaptability to different climates and soil types. From the European plum (Prunus domestica) to the Japanese plum (Prunus salicina) and several hybrids like the popular 'Santa Rosa' and 'Satsuma,' plum trees manifest a rich tapestry of genetic variation.

Cultural and Historical Significance: The cultivation of plum trees traces its roots back centuries, entwined within the historical and cultural narratives of many civilizations. The Chinese cultivated plums as early as 2,000 years ago, viewing them as symbols of longevity and perseverance. In Europe, plum trees found their way into gardens and orchards during Roman times and gained further popularity during the

Middle Ages. They hold significance not only as a food source but also in art, literature, and folklore, often representing vitality, abundance, and renewal.

Botanical Anatomy and Growth Habit: Plum trees typically boast a rounded, spreading canopy with glossy green leaves that turn vibrant hues of yellow and red in the fall. The distinctive flowers, ranging from white to various shades of pink, herald the arrival of spring with their captivating beauty and fragrance. The fruits, varying in size, shape, and color, ripen through the summer months, showcasing a spectrum from deep purple to golden yellow, red, or even green, depending on the cultivar.

Culinary and Nutritional Value: The fruits of plum trees offer a delectable blend of sweet and tart flavors, making them a sought-after ingredient in various cuisines. Whether enjoyed fresh, dried as prunes, or incorporated into jams, sauces, desserts, and beverages, plums impart a burst of flavors and essential nutrients. Rich in vitamins, antioxidants, and dietary fiber, plums contribute to overall health and well-being, promoting digestion, skin health, and immune function.

Adaptability and Cultivation: Plum trees exhibit a remarkable adaptability to diverse climates, thriving in temperate regions across the globe. However, specific cultivars may have preferences for certain environmental conditions, requiring adequate sunlight, well-draining soil, and proper care to maximize fruit production. Propagation methods include grafting, budding, or growing from seeds, with each method having its advantages and considerations.

plum trees stand as emblematic representatives of nature's bounty, offering not only luscious fruits but also beauty, resilience, and a rich tapestry of cultural and botanical significance. Their cultivation and appreciation span centuries, weaving through the fabric of human history and continuing to enchant and nourish generations to come.

1.2 Importance and Uses

The importance and uses of plum trees extend far beyond their delicious fruits, encompassing various facets of human life, culinary endeavors, cultural significance, and ecological roles.

Nutritional and Culinary Significance: Plums, derived from these trees, hold substantial nutritional value, brimming with vitamins, antioxidants, and dietary fiber. Whether consumed fresh, dried into prunes, or used in culinary creations, these fruits offer a delightful blend of flavors and textures. Their versatility in recipes, from jams and pies to savory dishes and beverages, adds depth and richness to cuisines worldwide.

Cultural and Symbolic Importance: Plum trees have embedded themselves within cultural symbolism across numerous societies. They often symbolize renewal, vitality, and abundance. In various cultures, plums are celebrated in rituals, art, literature, and festivals, carrying symbolic meanings tied to longevity, good fortune, and even artistic inspiration.

Horticultural and Ornamental Value: Beyond their fruits, plum trees exhibit stunning ornamental qualities. Their blossoms, adorning the branches in spring with hues ranging from delicate white to vibrant pink, make them prized ornamentals in gardens, parks, and landscapes. These trees contribute to the aesthetic appeal of environments, attracting pollinators and enhancing the beauty of the natural surroundings.

Economic and Agricultural Impact: Commercially, plum cultivation forms a significant aspect of the agricultural sector in many regions. The production and sale of plums and plum-related products contribute to local economies, providing employment opportunities and supporting the agricultural industry. Additionally, plum trees often serve as part of agroforestry systems, offering benefits such as erosion control and biodiversity enhancement.

Environmental and Ecological Role: Plum trees play a role in environmental conservation and ecosystem health. As deciduous trees, they contribute to carbon sequestration, improving air quality and mitigating the effects of climate change. Moreover, these trees provide habitats and food sources for various wildlife, including birds, insects, and small mammals, contributing to biodiversity preservation.

Medicinal and Health Benefits: Apart from their culinary uses, plums and their derivatives, like prunes, hold medicinal value. They aid in digestive health, containing compounds that support gut health and regulate digestion. Prunes, specifically, are known for their potential to alleviate constipation and promote overall digestive wellness.

The importance and uses of plum trees encompass a broad spectrum, from their nutritional and cultural significance to their role in horticulture, economics, ecology, and health. Beyond the delectable fruits they bear, these trees weave themselves intricately into the fabric of human existence, offering sustenance, beauty, and multifaceted contributions to our lives and the environment.

CHAPTER 2

Types of Plum Trees

2.1 Varieties and Species

Plum trees encompass a rich array of varieties and species, each with distinct characteristics, including fruit flavor, color, size, growth habits, and adaptability to varying climates. Here's an overview of some prominent varieties and species of plum trees:

1. European Plum (Prunus domestica):

- Renowned for its diverse cultivars like 'Stanley,' 'Italian Prune,' and 'Green Gage.'

- Typically features blue-purple fruits with yellow or greenish flesh.

- Often used for fresh consumption, drying into prunes, or making jams and preserves.

2. Japanese Plum (Prunus salicina):

- Includes popular varieties such as 'Santa Rosa,' 'Satsuma,' and 'Burbank.'

- Known for its larger, rounder fruits with a range of colors from red to yellow and even green.

- Tends to have juicier and sweeter fruits compared to European plums.

3. Damson Plum (Prunus domestica subsp. insititia):

- Smaller, oval-shaped fruits with
  a distinctive astringent flavor.

- Often used for making jams,
  jellies, and fruit-based spirits
  due to its high pectin content.

4. Mirabelle Plum (Prunus domestica subsp. syriaca):

- Small, yellow fruits with a
  sweet flavor, typically used for
  preserves and brandy
  production.

- Cultivated extensively in
  regions like Lorraine, France.

5. Cherry Plum (Prunus cerasifera):

- Known for its ornamental value
  and edible but smaller, cherry-
  sized fruits.

- Comes in various cultivars with different fruit colors, including red, yellow, and purple.

6. Hybrids and Crosses:

- Breeding efforts have led to numerous hybrid varieties, combining traits from different plum species for improved taste, disease resistance, and adaptability to specific climates.

- Examples include the 'Pluot' (plum-apricot hybrid) and 'Aprium' (apricot-plum hybrid), known for their unique flavors and textures.

7. Ornamental Plums:

- Some plum trees are primarily grown for their ornamental value, such as the purple-leaf plum (Prunus cerasifera 'Pissardii'), valued for its deep purple foliage and pink flowers rather than its fruit.

8. Wild Plums:

- Various wild species exist in different regions, often smaller in size and less cultivated but contributing to biodiversity and genetic diversity within the plum genus.

Each variety and species of plum tree offers a unique combination of characteristics, catering to different culinary preferences, climate conditions, and horticultural purposes. The diverse range of plum trees provides options for home gardeners, commercial orchards, and landscape designers, contributing to the richness of horticultural diversity and culinary delights.

2.2 Characteristics and Differences

The characteristics and differences among various types of plum trees encompass a range of factors, including fruit appearance, flavor, growth habits, and adaptability. Here's an exploration of these distinctions:

Fruit Appearance and Flavor:

- **European Plums:** These often feature a more oblong or oval shape with blue-purple skin and yellow or greenish flesh. They tend to have a slightly tart flavor, making them versatile for both fresh consumption and drying into prunes.

- **Japanese Plums:** Known for their larger, rounder fruits, they exhibit a diverse range of colors from red to yellow and even green. Japanese plums typically have juicier and sweeter fruits compared to European varieties.

- **Damson and Mirabelle Plums:** Damson plums are small and oval-shaped with an astringent flavor, primarily used for making jams and spirits. Mirabelle plums, on the other hand, are small, yellow, and have a sweeter taste, often utilized for preserves and brandy.

- **Cherry Plums:** These are smaller, cherry-sized fruits that come in various cultivars with different fruit colors, including red, yellow, and purple. They are often used for ornamental purposes but can be consumed fresh or used in cooking.

Growth Habits and Adaptability:

- **European and Japanese Plums:** These varieties typically have different growth habits; European plums tend to be more cold-hardy and adaptable to a wider range of climates, while Japanese plums may require warmer conditions and are often grown in more temperate regions.

- **Wild Plums:** Wild plum species may vary significantly in growth habits and adaptability based on their native regions. Some might thrive in specific climates or soil types, while others may be more resilient but produce smaller fruits.

Culinary Uses and Preferences:

- **European and Japanese Plums:** Differences in taste and texture make them suitable for various culinary applications. European plums are commonly used for drying into prunes, while Japanese plums are favored for fresh consumption due to their sweeter and juicier nature.

- **Hybrids and Cultivars:** Hybrid varieties, such as pluots or apriums, often aim to combine the best traits of different plum species, resulting in unique flavors, textures, and adaptability.

Ornamental Value:

- **Purple-Leaf Plum and Cherry Plums:** Some plum trees, like the purple-leaf plum or certain cherry plum cultivars, are grown primarily for their ornamental value. These trees may have smaller or less palatable fruits but exhibit striking foliage and blossoms, enhancing the aesthetic appeal of landscapes.

Understanding these characteristics and differences allows growers, gardeners, and enthusiasts to select plum tree varieties that align with their preferences, climate conditions, and intended purposes, whether for culinary delights, ornamental landscapes, or commercial cultivation.

2.3 Benefits of Plum Trees

Plum trees, renowned for their delicious fruits and ornamental beauty, offer a multitude of benefits, ranging from their nutritional value to their environmental contributions and aesthetic appeal.

Nutritional Benefits:

1. **Rich in Nutrients:** Plums are packed with essential nutrients like vitamins (A, C, K), minerals (potassium, magnesium), and dietary fiber, aiding in overall health.

2. **Antioxidant Properties:** High levels of antioxidants in plums help combat oxidative stress, reducing the risk of chronic diseases and promoting better immune function.

3. **Digestive Health:** The fiber content in plums supports digestive health by preventing constipation and promoting regular bowel movements.

Environmental Benefits:

1. **Ecosystem Support:** Plum trees serve as habitats for various insects, birds, and other wildlife, contributing to biodiversity.

2. **Soil Improvement:** Their root systems help prevent soil erosion and improve soil structure, enhancing fertility in the surrounding area.

3. **Air Quality:** Like other trees, plums contribute to cleaner air by absorbing carbon dioxide and releasing oxygen during photosynthesis.

Economic Benefits:

1. **Commercial Value:** Plum cultivation provides economic opportunities for farmers and businesses involved in the production and sale of fresh fruits, jams, juices, and other products.

2. **Landscaping and Ornamentation:** Ornamental plum varieties enhance property value and aesthetics in gardens, parks, and landscapes, attracting visitors and buyers.

Social Benefits:

1. **Community Engagement:** Plum trees, often found in community gardens or public spaces, foster community engagement and social interaction among residents.

2. **Educational Purposes:** They offer educational opportunities, especially in schools and educational institutions, teaching about agriculture, nutrition, and environmental conservation.

Culinary Benefits:

1. **Versatile Usage:** Plums can be eaten fresh, dried as prunes, or used in various culinary preparations like jams, sauces, pies, and desserts.

2. **Flavor Enhancement:** Their sweet and tangy flavor profile adds depth to dishes, making them a popular ingredient in both sweet and savory recipes.

Health and Wellness:

1. **Heart Health:** Regular consumption of plums is associated with reduced risk of heart-related issues due to their potassium content, which helps maintain healthy blood pressure levels.

2. **Weight Management:** The fiber in plums aids in weight management by promoting a feeling of fullness and regulating appetite.

The benefits of plum trees extend far beyond their delicious fruits. From their nutritional value and environmental contributions to economic, social, and even health-related advantages, these trees play a significant role in enhancing various aspects of our lives and the world around us. Whether in orchards, gardens, or urban landscapes, plum

trees stand as invaluable contributors
to our well-being and the
environment.

CHAPTER 3
Growing Plum Trees

3.1 Choosing the Right Location

Selecting the right location is crucial for successfully growing plum trees, ensuring optimal growth, fruit production, and overall tree health. Consider the following factors when choosing a suitable site for planting plum trees:

1. Climate Suitability:

- Plum trees thrive in various climates but generally prefer temperate regions with full sun exposure.

- Ensure the selected location aligns with the specific climatic requirements of the plum tree variety you're planting.

- Some varieties might require a certain number of chill hours (winter cold temperatures) to set fruit, so choose accordingly based on your region's climate.

2. Sunlight Requirements:

- Choose a site that receives ample sunlight, ideally at least 6 to 8 hours of direct sunlight daily. Full sun exposure promotes fruit production and ripening.

3. Soil Conditions:

- Plum trees prefer well-draining, loamy soil with a pH ranging between 5.5 and 6.5.

- Avoid waterlogged or heavy clay soils that can lead to root rot; adequate drainage is essential to prevent waterlogging.

4. Air Circulation:

- Good air circulation helps prevent fungal diseases. Avoid planting in low-lying areas or spots prone to frost pockets where cold air settles.

5. Protection from Wind:

- While some airflow is beneficial, excessive wind can damage the tree or its fruits. Consider planting near windbreaks or providing some protection if your area experiences strong winds.

6. Spacing and Positioning:

- Space plum trees appropriately based on their mature size. Standard plum trees generally require around 15 to 20 feet of space between each tree.

- Orient trees in an east-west direction to maximize sunlight exposure across the canopy.

7. Accessibility to Pollinators:

- Consider the proximity of plum trees to other fruit trees of compatible varieties for cross-pollination, as it can enhance fruit production. Some plum varieties are self-fertile, while others benefit from cross-pollination.

8. Urban Considerations:

- For urban settings, ensure adequate space for the tree's

root system to grow and access to sunlight despite potential nearby structures or shade.

Before planting, it's advisable to conduct a soil test to assess its pH and nutrient levels. Amend the soil as needed based on the test results to create an optimal environment for plum tree growth. Additionally, consider local climate patterns and microclimates within your area to choose a site that minimizes risks from late frosts or excessive heat, promoting healthy tree development and abundant fruit production.

3.2 Planting and Soil Requirements

When planting plum trees, meeting specific soil requirements and following proper planting procedures significantly contribute to their successful establishment and long-term health. Here's a guide on planting and soil requirements for plum trees:

1. Soil Preparation:

- Choose a well-draining site with fertile, loamy soil. Ensure the soil pH is between 5.5 and 6.5, which is optimal for plum tree growth.

- Prior to planting, clear the area of weeds, rocks, and debris. Loosen the soil to a depth of about 2 feet to encourage root penetration and establishment.

2. Selecting Healthy Trees:

- Purchase healthy, disease-free bare-root or container-grown plum trees from reputable

nurseries or garden centers.
Look for well-branched,
vigorous saplings with a strong
central leader (main trunk).

3. Planting Time:

- Plant plum trees during the
  dormant season, preferably in
  late winter or early spring
  before bud break. This timing
  encourages root establishment
  before active growth begins.

4. Planting Procedure:

- Dig a hole that's wide and deep
  enough to accommodate the
  root system without bending or
  crowding the roots. It should be
  slightly larger than the tree's
  root ball.

- Spread the roots evenly and
  position the tree in the center of

the hole at the same depth it was previously growing, with the graft union (if visible) above the soil line.

- Backfill the hole with the excavated soil, gently firming it around the roots to remove air pockets. Water thoroughly to settle the soil.

5. Mulching and Watering:

- Apply a 2 to 4-inch layer of organic mulch, like wood chips or compost, around the base of the tree without touching the trunk. Mulch helps retain soil moisture and regulates soil temperature.

- Water newly planted plum trees deeply immediately after planting to ensure proper hydration. Afterward, maintain regular watering, especially during dry periods, to keep the soil consistently moist but not waterlogged.

6. Fertilization and Pruning:

- Avoid fertilizing newly planted plum trees in the first year; allow them to establish roots before applying fertilizer.

- Pruning at planting should focus on removing damaged or crossing branches and maintaining a central leader, ensuring a well-balanced tree structure.

7. Support and Staking:

- Young trees might require staking to provide support against strong winds. Use flexible ties to secure the tree without causing damage to the trunk.

8. Careful Monitoring:

- Monitor the tree regularly for signs of stress, pests, or diseases. Proper care, including watering, mulching, and routine maintenance, is crucial during the initial years after planting.

By adhering to these planting procedures and soil requirements, you create an optimal environment for plum tree growth, fostering healthy root development and establishing a strong foundation for the tree's future productivity and longevity.

3.3 Watering and Maintenance

Watering and maintenance play pivotal roles in nurturing healthy plum trees, supporting their growth, fruit development, and overall vitality. Here's a comprehensive guide on watering and maintenance practices for plum trees:

1. Watering Guidelines:

- **Established Trees:** Once plum trees are established (usually after the first year), provide deep, thorough watering less frequently rather than frequent shallow watering. Aim for about 1 to 1.5 inches of water per week, adjusting based on weather conditions and soil moisture.

- **During Dry Periods:** Increase watering during hot, dry spells to maintain consistent soil moisture. Focus on watering the root zone, which extends beyond the tree's canopy.

- **Avoid Waterlogging:** Ensure proper drainage to prevent waterlogging, which can lead to root rot. Mulching helps retain soil moisture while allowing excess water to drain away.

2. Fertilization:

- **Early Years:** Refrain from fertilizing newly planted plum trees during their first year. In subsequent years, apply balanced fertilizer in early spring, after the danger of frost has passed, following package

instructions. Organic compost
can also be beneficial.

- **Avoid Excessive Nitrogen:**
Too much nitrogen can
promote excessive vegetative
growth at the expense of fruit
production. Use fertilizers with
balanced ratios (N-P-K)
suitable for fruit trees.

3. Pruning and Training:

- **Annual Pruning:** Prune plum
trees during the dormant season
to remove dead, damaged, or
diseased branches. Thin out
crowded growth to improve air
circulation and light
penetration.

- **Training:** Establish a central
leader structure for young plum
trees, removing competing

leaders and encouraging a well-balanced canopy.

4. Pest and Disease Management:

- **Monitoring:** Regularly inspect trees for signs of pests (such as aphids, plum curculio, or borers) and diseases (like brown rot, bacterial canker, or powdery mildew).

- **Integrated Pest Management (IPM):** Implement IPM strategies, which may include cultural practices, biological controls, and, if necessary, targeted pesticide applications, focusing on environmentally friendly approaches.

5. Winter Care:

- **Mulching:** Apply a layer of mulch around the base of the tree in late fall to insulate the soil and protect the roots from freezing temperatures.

- **Pruning:** Perform winter pruning to remove dead or damaged branches, promoting vigorous growth in the following spring.

6. Harvesting and Cleanliness:

- **Harvesting:** Pick plums when they reach full color and slight softness. Regularly harvest ripe fruits to prevent overloading branches and ensure better fruit quality.

- **Cleanup:** Remove fallen or rotting fruits promptly to prevent disease spread and attract pests.

7. Tree Support and Protection:

- **Staking:** Remove stakes and ties after the tree is established to prevent girdling or damage to the trunk.

- **Winter Protection:** Shield young trees from winter sunscald or rodent damage with tree guards or wraps.

Regular and attentive care, including proper watering, maintenance practices, pest and disease management, and seasonal tasks, contributes significantly to the health, vigor, and productivity of plum trees. Tailor care to the specific needs of your plum variety and local environmental conditions to ensure optimal growth and a bountiful harvest.

CHAPTER 4

Caring for Plum Trees

4.1 Pruning Techniques

Pruning is an essential aspect of caring for plum trees, contributing to their health, shape, and fruit production. Proper pruning techniques, timing, and considerations can make a significant difference in the tree's overall growth and yield. Here are some pruning techniques for plum trees:

1. Timing of Pruning:

- Prune plum trees during the dormant season, ideally in late winter or early spring before bud break. This timing minimizes stress on the tree and reduces the risk of disease transmission.

2. Tools and Sterilization:

- Use sharp, clean pruning tools such as hand pruners, loppers, and a pruning saw for larger branches. Ensure the tools are sanitized to prevent the spread of diseases between cuts. Use a disinfectant like rubbing alcohol or a diluted bleach solution.

3. Types of Pruning:

a. Thinning:

- Remove dead, diseased, or broken branches first. Then, thin out crowded areas to improve air circulation and sunlight penetration within the canopy. Aim for an open center or vase-shaped structure for optimal light exposure.

b. Heading Back:

- Use heading cuts to encourage lateral growth or control the height of the tree. Prune back the terminal branches to promote side branching, which can lead to more fruit-bearing wood.

c. Suckers and Watersprouts:

- Remove suckers (shoots growing from the base) and watersprouts (upright shoots within the canopy) to direct the tree's energy towards productive branches.

4. Pruning Techniques:

a. **Clean Cuts:** Make clean, angled cuts just outside the branch collar (the swollen area at the base of the branch) to aid in proper healing and minimize the risk of infection.

b. **Avoid Heavy Pruning:** Plum trees are susceptible to bacterial canker, so avoid heavy pruning, especially during the growing season, to reduce entry points for diseases.

c. **Pruning Young Trees:** Establish a strong framework by selectively pruning young trees to encourage a central leader and well-spaced lateral branches. Maintain a balanced canopy to support fruit production.

5. Disease Management:

- Apply pruning sealants or wound dressings only if diseases like bacterial canker are prevalent in your area. Otherwise, let the tree's natural healing process take place.

6. Post-Pruning Care:

- Clean up and remove all pruned materials from around the tree to prevent disease spread. Dispose of diseased branches away from the orchard area.

7. Continuous Monitoring:

- Regularly monitor the tree for any signs of disease, dieback, or pest infestation post-pruning. Promptly address any issues that arise.

Pruning practices should align with the overall health and growth goals for the plum tree, focusing on maintaining a balance between vegetative growth and fruit production while ensuring the tree's structural integrity. When done thoughtfully and correctly, pruning helps improve fruit quality, increase yield, and promote the long-term health of plum trees.

4.2 Pest and Disease Management

Managing pests and diseases is essential to maintain the health and productivity of plum trees. Implementing preventive measures and prompt intervention strategies can mitigate potential damage. Here are effective pest and disease management techniques for plum trees:

1. Pest Identification and Monitoring:

- Regularly inspect trees for signs of pests such as plum curculio, aphids, mites, borers, and caterpillars. Monitor foliage, branches, and fruit for unusual activity, damage, or infestations.

2. Cultural Practices:

- **Sanitation:** Keep the area around the tree clean by removing fallen leaves, fruit, and debris. This helps reduce shelter and breeding grounds for pests and diseases.

- **Proper Watering and Fertilization:** Avoid over-fertilizing as excessive nitrogen can make trees more susceptible to certain pests. Maintain proper soil moisture without waterlogging.

3. Biological Controls:

- Encourage natural predators and beneficial insects that prey on pests. For instance, ladybugs feed on aphids, providing natural pest control.

4. Horticultural Oils and Soaps:

- Use horticultural oils or insecticidal soaps to control aphids, mites, and scales. These products suffocate pests on contact without harming beneficial insects.

5. Pesticides:

- **Selective Pesticides:** If necessary, apply targeted pesticides specific to the pest and stage of infestation. Use pesticides labeled for plum trees and follow instructions carefully, ensuring proper timing and dosage.

- **Integrated Pest Management (IPM):** Adopt IPM strategies, combining various methods like cultural controls, biological controls, and pesticide applications in a systematic and environmentally friendly manner.

6. Disease Prevention:

- **Pruning Practices:** Practice proper pruning techniques, removing dead or diseased branches to prevent disease spread.

- **Fungicides:** Apply fungicides preventively if diseases like brown rot, bacterial canker, or powdery mildew are prevalent in your area. Follow label instructions and apply at the recommended times.

7. Timely Action:

- Take swift action at the first sign of pest or disease presence. Early intervention can prevent widespread infestations or infections.

8. Resistance Management:

- Rotate pesticide types to prevent the development of pesticide resistance in pests.

9. Consultation and Expert Advice:

- Seek guidance from local agricultural extension services, arborists, or experts to identify specific pests or diseases affecting plum trees in your region and determine appropriate control measures.

Combining preventive cultural practices, vigilant monitoring, and targeted intervention strategies tailored to the specific pest or disease challenges in your area can effectively manage and minimize the impact of pests and diseases on plum trees, promoting their health and productivity.

4.3 Fertilization Guidelines

Fertilization is essential for plum trees to maintain their vigor, promote healthy growth, and enhance fruit production. Proper fertilization practices, when tailored to the tree's needs and growth stages, can significantly benefit plum trees. Here are some fertilization guidelines for plum trees:

1. Soil Testing:

- Before applying fertilizers, conduct a soil test to assess nutrient levels, pH, and deficiencies. Soil testing helps determine the specific fertilizer needs of the plum trees.

2. Timing of Fertilization:

- **Established Trees:** Apply fertilizer in early spring, just before bud break, to support the tree's growth during the active growing season.

- **Young Trees:** Avoid fertilizing newly planted plum trees during their first year. Allow them to establish their root systems before applying fertilizer.

3. Balanced Fertilizers:

- Choose a balanced fertilizer formulated for fruit trees or a formulation with an N-P-K ratio appropriate for plum trees. A balanced fertilizer might have an equal or similar proportion of nitrogen (N), phosphorus (P), and potassium (K), such as 10-10-10 or 8-8-8.

- **Nitrogen Levels:** Plum trees generally do not require excessive nitrogen. Avoid over-application of nitrogen as it can lead to excessive vegetative growth at the expense of fruit production.

4. Application Techniques:

- **Broadcast Application:** Spread the fertilizer evenly around the drip line of the tree, which is the area under the outermost branches.

- **Deep Root Feeding:** Injecting fertilizer directly into the soil around the root zone can be an effective method for delivering nutrients to the tree's root system.

5. Quantity and Frequency:

- Apply fertilizer in accordance with the soil test recommendations and the specific needs of the tree. Over-fertilization can be detrimental.

- Splitting the total annual fertilizer dose into multiple applications throughout the growing season might be beneficial for the tree.

6. Organic Amendments:

- Incorporate organic materials such as compost, well-aged manure, or organic mulch around the base of the tree. These materials gradually release nutrients and improve soil structure.

7. Watering After Fertilization:

- Water the tree thoroughly after applying fertilizer to help dissolve and distribute the nutrients into the soil and encourage uptake by the roots.

8. Monitor Tree Response:

- Observe the tree's growth, foliage color, and fruit production. Adjust fertilizer applications based on the tree's response and annual soil tests.

Balanced fertilization, tailored to the specific needs of plum trees and guided by soil tests, promotes healthy growth, improves fruit quality, and supports the tree's overall health and resilience against environmental stressors. Regular monitoring and appropriate adjustments to the fertilization regimen contribute to the long-term success of plum tree cultivation.

CHAPTER 5

Harvesting and Utilizing Plums

5.1 Knowing When to Harvest

Knowing when to harvest plums is crucial to ensure they reach their peak ripeness, flavor, and sweetness. Plum varieties vary in color, size, and texture, so determining their readiness involves a combination of visual cues and touch. Here's a guide to help identify when plums are ready for harvest:

1. Color Changes:

- Check the plum's color. Depending on the variety,

plums can range from green to yellow, red, purple, or almost black when ripe. The exact color may vary based on the specific cultivar.

2. Firmness and Yielding to Touch:

- Gently squeeze the plum. Ripe plums should yield slightly to gentle pressure without being too soft or mushy. Overripe plums may feel overly soft and might have started to wrinkle.

3. Fullness and Size:

- Ripe plums tend to feel full and plump. They should have a round, full shape and not appear shriveled or underdeveloped.

4. Skin Texture:

- Check the skin for a slight bloom or dullness. Some plums develop a powdery coating known as a bloom when they are ripe, but this might not be present in all varieties.

5. Flavor and Aroma:

- Smell the plum near the stem end. Ripe plums often emit a sweet, fruity aroma. Taste-test a few fruits to ensure they have reached the desired sweetness and flavor.

6. Harvest Timeframes:

- Harvest times vary depending on the specific plum variety and local climate. Generally, plums ripen from late spring to late summer, but the timing can shift based on the cultivar and growing conditions.

- Some plums are clingstone, where the flesh sticks to the pit, and others are freestone, where the pit separates easily from the flesh. Freestone varieties are typically easier to harvest.

7. Multiple Harvests:

- For large plum trees or if the crop is vast, you might need to harvest in multiple sessions. Check the same tree or branch periodically for ripe fruit.

8. Weather Considerations:

- If heavy rains are forecast, it's advisable to harvest slightly early to prevent the fruit from becoming too waterlogged or splitting.

By paying attention to these visual, tactile, and taste cues, you can determine the optimal time to harvest plums, ensuring they are ripe, flavorful, and at their peak for consumption or preservation.

5.2 Storage and Preservation Tips

storing and preserving plums properly can extend their shelf life and allow you to enjoy them beyond the harvest season. Here are some tips for storing and preserving plums:

1. Short-Term Storage:

- Place ripe plums in a single layer in the refrigerator, ideally in the crisper drawer or a shallow container. They can remain fresh for about 3 to 5 days when refrigerated.

2. Handling Ripe Plums:

- Handle ripe plums gently to avoid bruising or damaging the skin, which can lead to quicker spoilage.

3. Freezing Plums:

- Wash and dry plums thoroughly. Remove pits and slice or chop the fruit as desired.

- Spread the prepared plums on a baking sheet lined with parchment paper, ensuring they don't touch each other, and freeze them until firm.

- Once frozen, transfer the plums to airtight containers or freezer bags. They can be stored in the freezer for up to several months.

4. Canning and Preserving:

- Plums can be canned or made into jams, preserves, or fruit sauces. Follow safe canning practices and use appropriate recipes to ensure proper preservation and avoid spoilage.

- High-acid fruits like plums are generally suitable for water bath canning methods.

5. Drying Plums (Prunes):

- To make prunes, slice ripe plums in half and remove the pits. Arrange the halves on drying racks or trays, ensuring good airflow.

- Dry the plums in a dehydrator or an oven set to its lowest temperature, aiming for a chewy texture. It can take 24 to 48 hours or longer depending

on the method and humidity
levels.

- Store dried plums in airtight
  containers in a cool, dry place
  for several months.

6. Fruit Leather:

- Puree ripe plums in a blender
  and spread the mixture thinly
  on parchment-lined trays or
  baking sheets.

- Dry the puree in an oven or a
  food dehydrator until it
  becomes a pliable, leathery
  consistency.

- Cut the fruit leather into strips
  and store in airtight containers
  or wrap individually for later
  consumption.

7. Pickling or Fermenting:

- Plums can also be pickled or fermented to create tangy and flavorful condiments. Explore recipes for plum chutneys or pickled plums.

Proper storage methods and preservation techniques allow you to enjoy plums well beyond their fresh harvest season. Whether refrigerating, freezing, canning, drying, or using them in creative recipes, these methods can help you make the most of your plum harvest.

5.3 Culinary Uses and Recipes

Plums offer a delightful range of culinary possibilities, from sweet desserts to savory dishes and tangy condiments. Here are some culinary uses and recipes showcasing the versatility of plums:

1. Desserts:

- **Plum Tart:** Prepare a simple tart with sliced plums arranged on a pastry base, sprinkled with sugar and spices, then baked until golden.

- **Plum Crumble:** Combine sliced plums with sugar and cinnamon, top with a crumbly mixture of oats, flour, butter, and sugar, and bake until the topping is golden and crispy.

2. Preserves and Jams:

- **Plum Jam:** Cook plums with sugar and a touch of lemon juice until they reach a jam-like consistency. Store in sterilized jars for later use as a spread or topping.

3. Savory Dishes:

- **Grilled Plums:** Halve plums, remove the pits, and grill them until caramelized. Serve as a side dish with grilled meats or as a topping for salads.

- **Plum Sauce:** Cook plums with vinegar, sugar, and spices to create a tangy and sweet sauce ideal for glazing roasted or grilled meats.

4. Beverages:

- **Plum Smoothie:** Blend ripe plums with yogurt, honey, and ice for a refreshing and nutritious smoothie.

- **Plum-infused Water:** Add sliced plums to a pitcher of

water for a subtly flavored and refreshing drink.

5. Baking:

- **Plum Bread:** Incorporate chopped plums into a bread batter for a moist and flavorful bread loaf.

6. Salad Additions:

- **Plum Salad:** Combine fresh plums with greens, nuts, cheese, and a vinaigrette dressing for a vibrant and flavorful salad.

7. Chutneys and Pickles:

- **Spiced Plum Chutney:** Cook plums with spices, vinegar, sugar, and onions to create a tangy and spicy condiment perfect with cheese or roasted meats.

Recipe: Plum Crisp/Crumble:

Ingredients:

- 4 cups sliced plums

- 1/2 cup granulated sugar (adjust according to plum sweetness)

- 1 teaspoon ground cinnamon

- 1 cup old-fashioned oats

- 1/2 cup all-purpose flour

- 1/2 cup brown sugar

- 1/2 cup unsalted butter (cold and cubed)

- Pinch of salt

Instructions:

1. Preheat oven to 375°F (190°C). Grease a baking dish.

2. In a bowl, toss sliced plums with granulated sugar and cinnamon. Transfer to the prepared baking dish.

3. In another bowl, combine oats, flour, brown sugar, and salt. Add the cubed butter and rub it into the mixture until it resembles coarse crumbs.

4. Spread the crumbly mixture over the plums in the baking dish.

5. Bake for 35-40 minutes or until the top is golden brown and the plum juices are bubbling.

6. Allow it to cool slightly before serving. Enjoy warm with ice cream or whipped cream.

Plums' sweet-tart flavor and versatility make them a delightful addition to various dishes, whether as the star ingredient in desserts, a tangy addition to savory dishes, or a flavorful component in condiments and beverages. Experiment with these recipes or create your own to explore the culinary potential of plums!

CHAPTER 6

Troubleshooting Common Issues

6.1 Identifying Problems

Identifying and diagnosing issues with plum trees is essential for prompt intervention and maintaining tree health. Here are common problems and their signs that may affect plum trees:

1. Pests:

- **Plum Curculio:** Leaves small crescent-shaped scars or holes in developing fruits.

- **Aphids:** Clustered on new growth, causing leaf curling, distortion, and sticky honeydew residue.

- **Plum Moth Larvae:** Enter fruits, leaving tunnels and causing fruit drop or premature ripening.

- **Borers:** Presence of small holes in the trunk or branches, frass (sawdust-like residue), and weakened branches.

2. Diseases:

- **Brown Rot:** Causes brown, mushy spots on fruits, often with grayish spores in humid conditions.

- **Bacterial Canker:** Shows as sunken lesions on branches or trunk, often exuding gum or oozing dark sap.

- **Powdery Mildew:** Powdery white spots on leaves and shoots, leading to distorted growth.

3. Environmental Stressors:

- **Fruit Drop:** Excessive fruit drop might result from poor pollination, water stress, or nutrient deficiencies.

- **Leaf Wilting or Yellowing:** Indicative of overwatering, underwatering, or root issues.

- **Sunscald:** Sun-exposed bark can develop cracks or lesions due to extreme heat, leading to cankers.

4. Nutritional Deficiencies:

- **Iron Deficiency:** Yellowing between leaf veins, called

chlorosis, indicating lack of iron.

- **Nitrogen Deficiency:** Stunted growth, yellowing of older leaves, and reduced fruit production.

5. Mechanical Damage:

- **Branch Breakage:** Weak unions or overcrowded branches leading to breakage, especially during storms.

- **Trunk Damage:** Cuts, wounds, or physical injuries to the trunk affecting overall tree health.

6. Poor Pollination:

- **Low Fruit Set:** Insufficient pollination can result in low fruit set, leading to reduced yield.

7. Other Factors:

- **Weed Competition:**
  Overgrown weeds competing
  for water and nutrients around
  the tree.

- **Improper Pruning:** Incorrect
  pruning practices causing
  stress, improper growth, or
  disease susceptibility.

Regular monitoring, observation, and
understanding of these signs and
symptoms enable early intervention
and appropriate remedies to address
the issues and ensure the continued
health and productivity of plum trees.

6.2 Solutions and Troubleshooting

Addressing issues with plum trees
involves specific solutions tailored to

each problem. Here are troubleshooting tips and solutions for common plum tree issues:

1. Pests:

- **Plum Curculio or Moth Larvae:** Apply insecticides labeled for plum trees at the appropriate times following local extension service recommendations. Keep the area clean to reduce overwintering sites.

- **Aphids:** Use insecticidal soap or horticultural oils to control small infestations. Encourage natural predators like ladybugs or lacewings.

- **Borers:** Physically remove affected branches or use insecticides if infestation is severe. Maintain tree health to prevent vulnerability to borers.

2. Diseases:

- **Brown Rot:** Remove infected fruits and prune affected branches during the dormant season. Apply fungicides during bud break if necessary. Ensure good air circulation around the tree.

- **Bacterial Canker:** Prune infected branches well below the affected area, disinfecting tools between cuts. Copper-based fungicides can help prevent spread.

- **Powdery Mildew:** Apply fungicides labeled for powdery mildew control. Improve air circulation and reduce humidity around the tree.

3. Environmental Stressors:

- **Fruit Drop:** Improve pollination by introducing pollinator-attracting plants nearby. Maintain consistent watering and fertilization practices.

- **Leaf Issues:** Adjust watering to maintain consistent moisture levels. Address root problems, if any, and ensure proper drainage.

- **Sunscald:** Protect the trunk with tree wraps or paint to prevent direct sunlight damage.

4. Nutritional Deficiencies:

- **Iron or Nitrogen Deficiency:** Apply appropriate fertilizers or nutrient supplements based on soil test results. Follow recommended dosages to avoid over-fertilization.

5. Mechanical Damage:

- **Branch Breakage:** Prune back overcrowded branches, especially those with weak unions. Stake or brace vulnerable branches during storms.

- **Trunk Damage:** Clean and protect wounds with pruning paint or sealant to prevent infections and encourage healing.

6. Poor Pollination:

- **Introduce Pollinators:** Plant flowers or flowering shrubs to attract bees and other pollinators. Hand pollination can be an option for small trees.

7. Other Factors:

- **Weed Competition:** Mulch around the tree to suppress weed growth and reduce competition for nutrients and water.

- **Proper Pruning:** Educate yourself on correct pruning techniques or seek guidance from a professional arborist to avoid stress or disease susceptibility.

prevention is often the best strategy. Maintaining tree health through proper cultural practices, regular inspection, and timely intervention can prevent many issues from arising in the first place. If problems persist or are severe, consulting with local arborists or extension services for personalized guidance can be immensely helpful in addressing specific plum tree issues.